PURE DIET COOKBOOK

FOR ADULTS

Quick and Easy-to-Prepare Recipes For Seniors with Chewing and Swallowing Difficulty

By

ALICIA TRAVIS

Copyright © 2024 by Alicia Travis

All rights reserved. No part of this publication may be reproduced, distributed, or transmitted in any form or by any means, including photocopying, recording, or other electronic or mechanical methods, without the prior written permission of the publisher. It is illegal to copy this book, distribute it or even post it on any website without permission.

TABLE OF CONTENT

INTRODUCTION 5
CHAPTER 1: UNDERSTANDING PUREE DIET 7
    1.1 What is a Puree Diet? 7
    1.2 Who Might Benefit from a Puree Diet? 7
    1.3 Importance of Nutritional Balance in the Puree Diet 9
CHAPTER 2: GETTING STARTED 13
    2.1 Necessary Kitchen Tools and Equipment 13
    2.2 Basic Cooking Techniques for Pureeing 14
    2.3 Tips for Preparing Delicious Pureed Meals 15
    2.4 Choosing Ingredients for Purees 17
    2.5 Thickening and Thinning Purees 18
    2.6 Flavor Boosters for Purees 18
    2.7 Pureeing Techniques 19
    2.8 Storing and Reheating Pureed Foods 20
CHAPTER 3: PUREE-FRIENDLY RECIPES FOR ADULTS 21
BREAKFAST RECIPES 21
    Green Smoothie Puree 22
    Creamy Berry Oatmeal Puree 23
    Vegetable Breakfast Puree 24
    Creamy Banana Nut Breakfast Puree 25
    Pumpkin Spice Breakfast Puree 26
    Creamy Coconut Mango Chia Pudding Puree 27
    Creamy Spinach and Feta Breakfast Puree 28
    Soft Blueberry Pancakes with Yogurt Sauce 29
    Soft Breakfast Casserole with Sweet Potatoes and Turkey 30
    Creamy Pumpkin Breakfast Smoothie 31
    Soft Baked Apples with Yogurt and Granola 32
    Soft Scrambled Tofu with Spinach and Cheese 33
    Banana Peanut Butter Smoothie 34
    Soft French Toast with Berries and Honey 35
    Creamy Mango Banana Smoothie Bowl 36
    Soft Boiled Eggs with Toast Soldiers 37
    Creamy Blueberry Banana Smoothie 38
    Soft Baked Oatmeal with Berries 39

Soft Ricotta Pancakes with Berry Compote..40
Burrito with Scrambled Eggs and Avocado...41
Creamy Banana Oatmeal..42
Silken Smoothie..43
Green Smoothie Bowl..44
Soft Scrambled Eggs with Herbs...45
Banana Yogurt Pancakes..46

HEALING SOUPS AND BROTHS RECIPES...47
Creamy Carrot Ginger Soup..48
Spinach and Avocado Soup...49
Broccoli and Cauliflower Puree...50
Creamy Mushroom Soup..51
Sweet Potato and Coconut Soup... 52
Pea and Mint Puree...53
Creamy Asparagus Soup...54
Tomato and Red Pepper Bisque..55
Lentil and Coconut Curry Soup..56
Creamy Cauliflower and Leek Soup... 57
Smooth and Creamy Mashed Potatoes..58
Garlic Infused Cauliflower Mash...59
Creamed Spinach with Nutmeg..60
Pureed Carrots with Ginger..61
Velvety Pumpkin Puree..62
Beetroot and Potato Mash...63
Zucchini and Basil Puree..64
Broccoli and Cheese Puree...65
Sweet Potato and Coconut Puree..66
Creamy Asparagus and Potato Puree..67

DESSERT RECIPES...68
Cinnamon-Spiced Sweet Potato Mash...69
Velvety Chocolate Avocado Mousse..69
Ginger-Infused Carrot Cake Puree..70
Soothing Apple Cinnamon Sauce..70
Minty Pea and Coconut Puree.. 71
Creamy Banana Almond Butter Puree.. 71
Creamy Vanilla Bean Pear Puree...72

Soothing Pumpkin Spice Puree..72
Cozy Maple Cinnamon Butternut Squash Mash.......................................73
Soothing Chamomile Infused Peach Puree..73

HEALTHY AND TASTY SNACK RECIPES................................... 74
Avocado and White Bean Dip...74
Sweet Potato and Carrot Hummus..75
Beet and Greek Yogurt Dip...76
Spinach and White Bean Puree...77
Mango and Banana Smoothie...78

CONCLUSION... 79

INTRODUCTION

In the area of dietary interventions, the puree diet stands as a versatile approach with a rich history and diverse applications. This dietary regimen, characterized by its texture and consistency, has been a cornerstone in culinary and healthcare practices for centuries. While it may seem simple on the surface, the puree diet carries profound significance for individuals across various age groups and health conditions.

This cookbook aims to look deep into the puree diet, unraveling its origins, defining its essence, and shedding light on its potential benefits. From its humble beginnings to its modern-day applications, we will journey through the annals of history to understand how this dietary modality has evolved and adapted to meet the ever-changing needs of adults seeking nourishment and healing.

The concept of pureed foods finds its origins intertwined with the evolution of culinary practices and medical interventions. Historically, pureeing food has been utilized to cater to various dietary needs, ranging from infants transitioning to solid foods to individuals with dysphagia, a condition characterized by difficulty in swallowing.

Ancient civilizations such as the Egyptians and Romans utilized rudimentary methods to puree foods, often employing mortar and pestle to create mashed or blended concoctions. However, it was not until the Renaissance period that the concept of pureed foods gained recognition as a therapeutic tool.

Physicians like Paracelsus advocated for the consumption of finely mashed foods for patients with digestive ailments, laying the groundwork for the integration of pureed diets into medical practice.

As medical understanding advanced, particularly in the fields of nutrition and gastroenterology, the puree diet emerged as a structured dietary regimen. In the 20th century, with the advent of industrialization and technological innovations, the production of pureed foods became more streamlined, enabling mass production and distribution to cater to diverse dietary requirements.

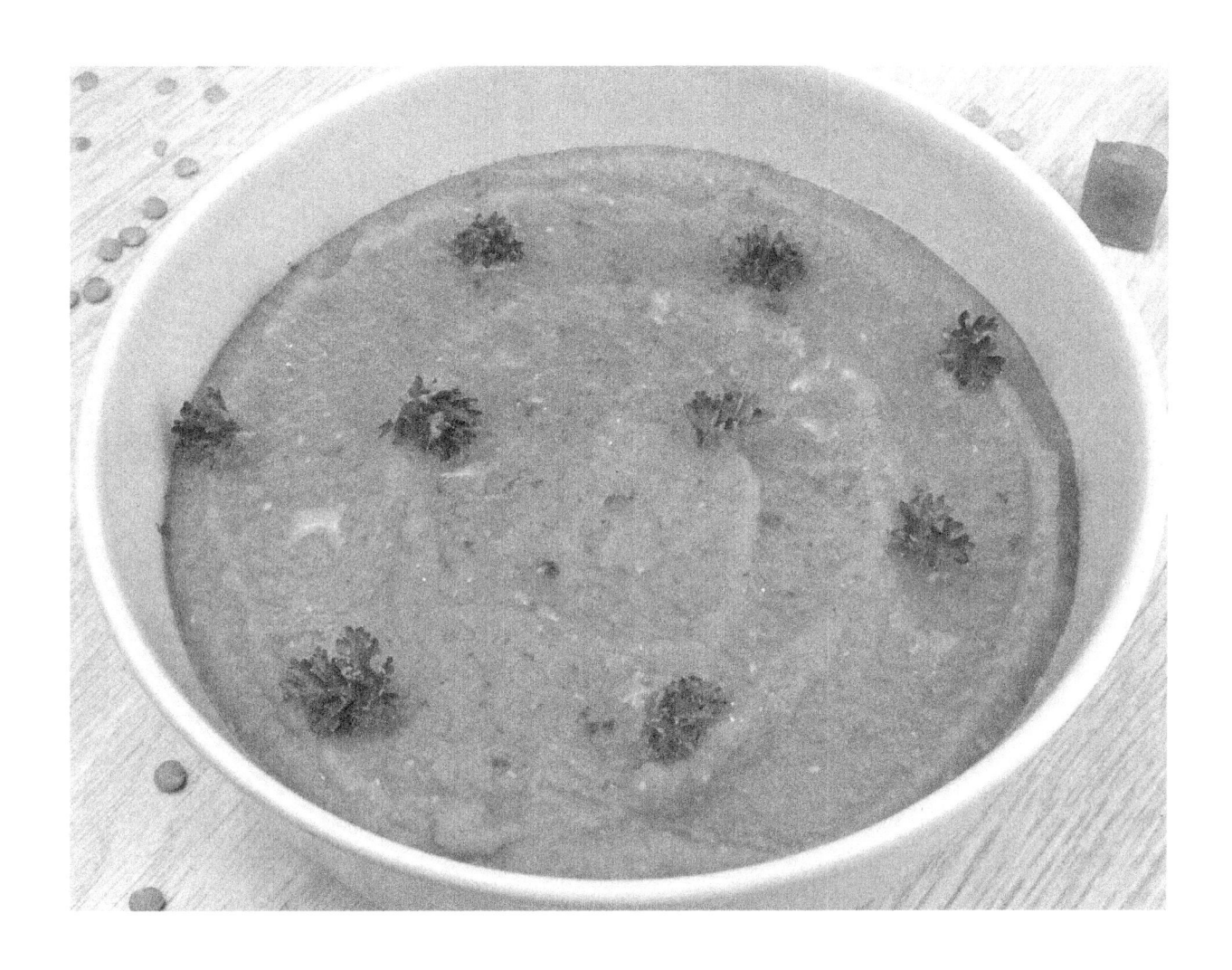

CHAPTER 1: UNDERSTANDING PUREE DIET

1.1 What is a Puree Diet?

At its core, the puree diet revolves around the consumption of foods that have been blended or processed into a smooth, homogeneous consistency. Unlike solid foods, which require chewing and swallowing, pureed foods are rendered into a form that can be easily ingested and digested by adults with difficulty chewing or swallowing.

A puree diet, also known as a blenderized or soft food diet, involves the consumption of foods that have been processed into a smooth, uniform consistency. The process of pureeing entails blending solid foods with liquid (such as water, broth, or milk) until they reach a smooth texture, devoid of any solid particles.

The primary objective of a puree diet is to facilitate easier swallowing and digestion, making it suitable for adults with various medical conditions affecting their ability to chew or swallow solid foods. While the specific texture and composition of pureed foods may vary depending on individual needs and dietary restrictions, common examples include mashed potatoes, blended soups, fruit smoothies, and pureed meats.

While the term "puree" may evoke images of baby food or hospital meals, the reality is that this dietary approach encompasses a wide range of culinary possibilities. From creamy soups and silky smoothies to decadent desserts and savory spreads, pureed foods can be as diverse and flavorful as their solid counterparts, offering a wealth of options for those following this dietary regimen.

1.2 Who Might Benefit from a Puree Diet?

The puree diet serves as a valuable resource for adults facing various challenges related to chewing, swallowing, or digesting solid foods. While its primary audience may include infants transitioning to solid foods and elderly individuals experiencing age-related changes in swallowing function, the benefits of the puree diet extend far beyond these demographic groups. Some of the key beneficiaries of the puree diet include:

Dysphagia Patients: One of the primary beneficiaries of the puree diet is individuals with dysphagia, a medical condition characterized by difficulty swallowing. Dysphagia can arise from a multitude of causes, including neurological disorders such as stroke or Parkinson's disease, structural abnormalities in the throat or esophagus, or muscular weakness due to aging or illness,which renders swallowing difficult or painful. For these individuals, consuming solid foods can pose a significant risk of choking or aspiration, making pureed foods a safer and more practical alternative.

Geriatric Population: Aging often brings about changes in oral health, muscle strength, and coordination, predisposing elderly individuals to swallowing difficulties. A puree diet addresses the unique nutritional needs of seniors, ensuring adequate nourishment without compromising safety.

Patients Recovering from Surgery: Surgical interventions, particularly those involving the oral or gastrointestinal tract, may necessitate temporary adherence to a puree diet during the recovery phase. Pureed foods minimize stress on surgical sites and promote healing without impeding nutritional intake.

Infants and Toddlers: During the transition from breastfeeding or formula feeding to solid foods, infants and toddlers may encounter challenges in chewing and swallowing. Pureed baby foods serve as an essential introduction to solid foods, facilitating the development of oral motor skills and taste preferences.

Individuals with Oral or Dental Issues: Dental problems, oral injuries, or conditions such as temporomandibular joint (TMJ) disorders can hinder the mastication process, making it uncomfortable or impossible to consume solid foods. Pureed diets alleviate strain on the oral cavity, allowing individuals to meet their nutritional requirements while undergoing dental treatment or rehabilitation.

In addition to the aforementioned conditions, the puree diet may also benefit individuals with certain medical conditions or dietary restrictions that necessitate a soft or easily digestible diet. This includes patients recovering from oral or maxillofacial surgery, individuals undergoing treatment for conditions such as oral cancer or temporomandibular joint (TMJ) disorders, and those with gastrointestinal disorders such as gastroparesis or inflammatory bowel disease (IBD). For these individuals, the puree diet provides a means of obtaining essential nutrients and calories without exacerbating their underlying health issues.

Furthermore, the puree diet can be a valuable tool for caregivers and healthcare professionals seeking to ensure adequate nutrition for their patients or loved ones. By offering a diverse array of pureed foods that are both nutritious and appetizing, caregivers can help maintain the health and well-being of those under their care while accommodating their specific dietary needs and preferences.

1.3 Importance of Nutritional Balance in the Puree Diet

While the primary goal of the puree diet is to ensure safe and efficient swallowing, it is imperative to underscore the critical role of nutritional balance within this dietary framework. Despite the homogenized texture of pureed foods, maintaining optimal nutrition remains paramount to sustaining overall health and vitality. Achieving nutritional balance on a puree diet requires careful consideration of factors such as nutrient density, variety, and portion sizes to meet the unique needs of each individual.

Nutrient Density

One of the key considerations when planning a puree diet is the nutrient density of the foods consumed. Nutrient density refers to the concentration of essential nutrients, such as vitamins, minerals, protein, and fiber, relative to the total calories provided by a food or meal. Choosing nutrient-dense foods ensures that individuals receive maximum nutritional benefit from their diet without consuming excessive calories or empty carbohydrates.

When selecting foods for pureeing, it is important to prioritize those that are rich in essential nutrients and contribute to overall health and well-being. This includes incorporating a variety of fruits, vegetables, lean proteins, and whole grains into pureed meals to ensure a balanced intake of vitamins, minerals, and macronutrients. For example, pureed fruits such as berries, bananas, and mangoes provide a rich source of vitamins C and K, potassium, and fiber, while pureed vegetables like spinach, carrots, and sweet potatoes offer an abundance of vitamins A and C, folate, and antioxidants.

In addition to fruits and vegetables, lean proteins are an essential component of a nutritious puree diet, providing the building blocks for muscle repair and growth, immune function, and hormone production. Sources of lean protein suitable for pureeing include cooked poultry, fish, tofu, legumes, and dairy products such as Greek yogurt or cottage cheese. By incorporating a variety of protein-rich foods into pureed meals, individuals can meet their daily protein requirements and support optimal health and vitality.

Variety

Incorporating a diverse range of foods into the puree diet is essential for ensuring adequate intake of essential nutrients and preventing nutrient deficiencies. Variety not only enhances the nutritional quality of meals but also helps to stimulate the appetite and prevent dietary boredom, which can be common challenges for individuals following a restricted diet.

When planning pureed meals, it is important to include a variety of colors, flavors, and textures to appeal to the senses and promote enjoyment of eating. This may involve experimenting with different combinations of fruits, vegetables, proteins, and grains to create flavorful and visually appealing pureed dishes. For example, a pureed vegetable soup made with vibrant ingredients such as tomatoes, bell peppers, carrots, and kale not only provides a wealth of vitamins and minerals but also tantalizes the taste buds with its rich flavor and velvety texture.

In addition to incorporating a variety of whole foods into pureed meals, it is also important to consider the use of herbs, spices, and other flavor enhancers to elevate the taste and aroma of dishes. Fresh herbs such as basil, cilantro, and mint can add depth and complexity to pureed soups and sauces, while spices such as cinnamon, cumin, and ginger can impart warmth and flavor to pureed desserts and smoothies. By experimenting with different flavor combinations and seasoning techniques, individuals can create delicious and satisfying pureed meals that cater to their unique tastes and preferences.

Portion Sizes

While the puree diet offers flexibility in terms of food choices and meal options, it is important to pay attention to portion sizes to avoid overeating and maintain a healthy weight. Portion control plays a crucial role in managing caloric intake and preventing excessive weight gain, which can contribute to a host of health issues such as obesity, diabetes, and heart disease.

When serving pureed meals, it is helpful to use measuring cups, spoons, or kitchen scales to portion out appropriate serving sizes based on individual calorie and nutrient needs. This may involve consulting with a healthcare professional or registered dietitian to determine personalized portion guidelines that take into account factors such as age, gender, activity level, and medical history.

In addition to controlling portion sizes, it is also important to practice mindful eating habits such as eating slowly, chewing thoroughly, and paying attention to hunger and fullness cues. By savoring each bite and listening to the body's signals, individuals can enjoy their meals more fully and avoid overeating or feeling deprived.

1.4 The essential components of nutritional balance in the puree diet:

1. Macronutrient Composition

Carbohydrates: Carbohydrates serve as the primary energy source in the diet, providing fuel for bodily functions and physical activity. In the puree diet, complex carbohydrates from whole grains, legumes, and starchy vegetables can be incorporated into blended dishes such as pureed lentil soup or mashed sweet potatoes.

Proteins: Proteins are indispensable for tissue repair, immune function, and muscle maintenance. Pureed meats, poultry, fish, tofu, legumes, and dairy products serve as rich sources of protein, ensuring adequate intake to support growth and healing.

Fats: While fats often contribute to flavor and satiety, they also play a crucial role in nutrient absorption and hormone production. Incorporating healthy fats from sources such as avocados, nuts, seeds, and olive oil into pureed dishes enhances both taste and nutritional value.

2. Micronutrient Density

Vitamins: Essential vitamins, such as vitamin A, vitamin C, vitamin D, and various B vitamins, are vital for numerous physiological processes, including vision, immunity, and energy metabolism. Pureed fruits and vegetables, particularly brightly colored varieties, supply an array of vitamins, ensuring comprehensive micronutrient support.

Minerals: Minerals such as calcium, iron, magnesium, and potassium play pivotal roles in bone health, oxygen transport, muscle function, and electrolyte balance. Incorporating mineral-rich ingredients like leafy greens, nuts, seeds, and dairy products into pureed recipes promotes optimal mineral intake.

3. Fiber Content

Fiber, though often overlooked in pureed diets, remains crucial for digestive health, satiety, and blood sugar regulation. While the blending process may reduce the fiber content of foods, incorporating fiber-rich ingredients such as fruits, vegetables, whole grains, and legumes into pureed dishes can help mitigate potential deficiencies.

4. Hydration Status

Maintaining adequate hydration is paramount, especially for individuals with dysphagia or those at risk of dehydration. Pureed soups, smoothies, and thin purees can contribute to overall fluid intake, supplementing the body's hydration needs alongside water and other beverages.

5. Texture Modification

Texture modification is a cornerstone of the puree diet, as it ensures safe swallowing while preserving nutritional integrity. Graduating from smoother purees to slightly textured or minced foods as tolerated can facilitate the transition back to solid foods while promoting oral motor skills and sensory stimulation.

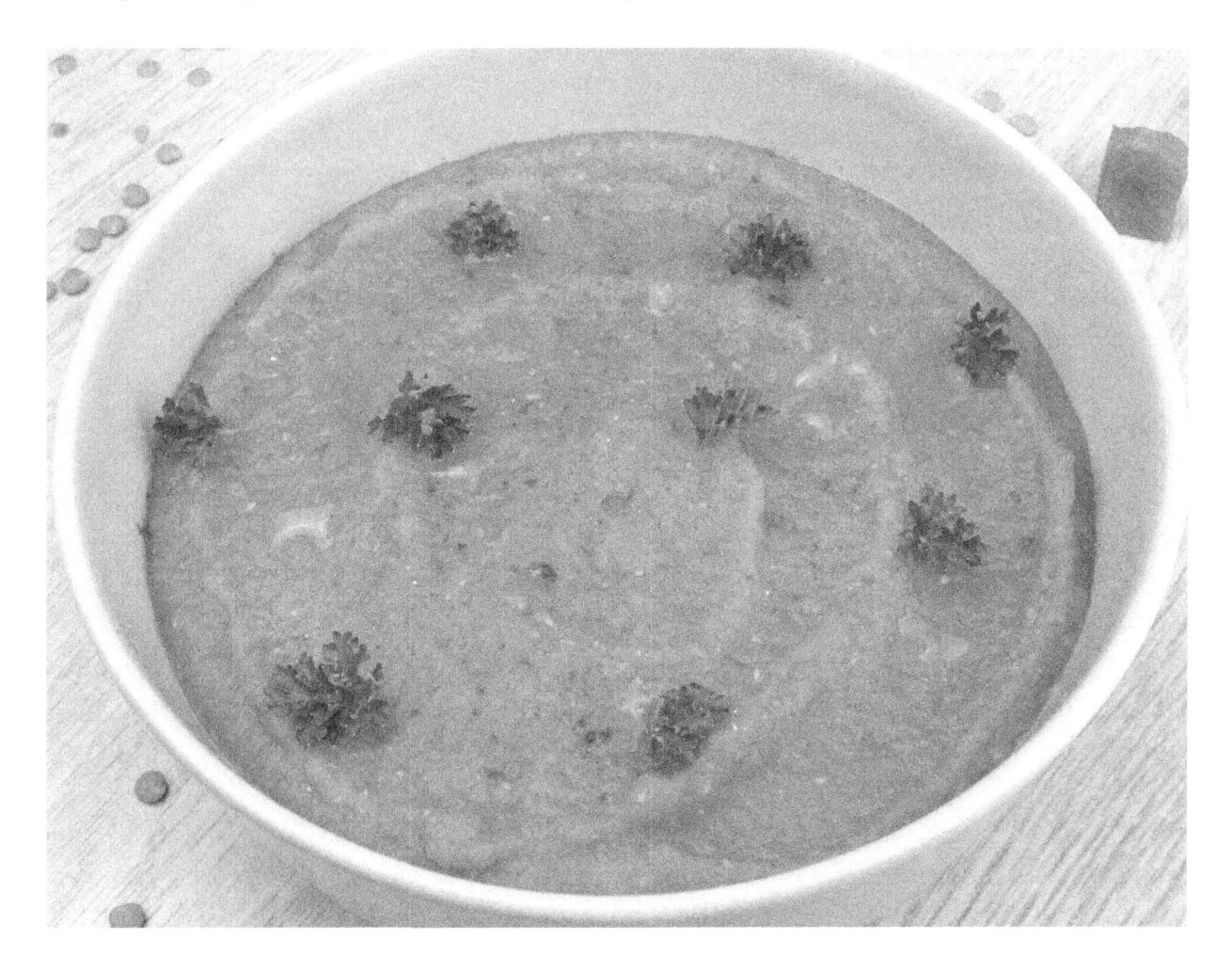

CHAPTER 2: GETTING STARTED

Whether you're just starting out or looking to refine your skills, understanding the necessary kitchen tools and equipment, mastering basic cooking techniques for pureeing, and learning tips for preparing delicious pureed meals are essential steps towards becoming proficient in this cuisine area.

2.1 Necessary Kitchen Tools and Equipment

Before diving into the world of pureed cooking, it's important to have the right tools and equipment at your disposal. Here's a comprehensive list of what you'll need:

Blender or Food Processor: A high-quality blender or food processor is the cornerstone of pureed cooking. It's essential for breaking down solid ingredients into smooth, creamy textures. Look for a model with sharp blades and variable speed settings for optimal results.

Strainer or Sieve: A fine-mesh strainer or sieve is necessary for removing any lumps or fibers from your purees, resulting in a smoother consistency.

Rubber Spatula: A rubber spatula is handy for scraping down the sides of your blender or food processor to ensure that all ingredients are thoroughly blended.

Vegetable Peeler: A vegetable peeler is essential for removing the skins from fruits and vegetables before pureeing them.

Cutting Board and Knife: A sturdy cutting board and sharp knife are indispensable for chopping and preparing ingredients before pureeing.

Measuring Cups and Spoons: Accurate measurement is key in cooking, so make sure you have a set of measuring cups and spoons on hand for precise ingredient amounts.

Pots and Pans: While not exclusively for pureed cooking, having a variety of pots and pans in different sizes is essential for preparing ingredients before pureeing or cooking pureed dishes on the stovetop.

Storage Containers: Having a selection of airtight storage containers will allow you to store leftover purees or prepare batches in advance for future use.

Immersion Blender (Optional): An immersion blender, also known as a hand blender, can be a convenient alternative to a traditional blender or food processor, especially for smaller batches or when working directly in pots or pans.

Now that you have the necessary tools and equipment, let's move on to mastering basic cooking techniques for pureeing.

2.2 Basic Cooking Techniques for Pureeing

Pureeing is a cooking method that involves blending or processing ingredients into a smooth, uniform consistency. While it may seem straightforward, there are some essential techniques to master to achieve perfect purees every time:

Preparing Ingredients: Start by washing and peeling any fruits or vegetables you plan to use in your puree. Remove any seeds, pits, or tough stems as needed. For meats or other proteins, trim away any excess fat or gristle.

Chopping: Once your ingredients are prepped, chop them into small, uniform pieces to ensure even cooking and easier blending. For harder ingredients like root vegetables or meats, smaller pieces will help speed up the cooking process.

Cooking: Depending on the recipe, you may need to cook your ingredients before pureeing them. This can be done by boiling, steaming, roasting, or sautéing, depending on the desired flavor and texture. Cooking also helps soften ingredients, making them easier to blend.

Blending: Transfer your cooked ingredients to a blender or food processor and blend until smooth. Start on a low speed and gradually increase to high for the smoothest consistency. Use a rubber spatula to scrape down the sides as needed to ensure all ingredients are evenly blended.

Straining (Optional): For an extra-smooth puree, strain it through a fine-mesh strainer or sieve to remove any remaining lumps or fibers. This step is especially important for achieving a velvety texture in soups or sauces.

Seasoning: Taste your puree and adjust the seasoning as needed with salt, pepper, herbs, or spices. Remember that pureed foods can sometimes require more seasoning than their whole counterparts, as blending can dull the flavor intensity.

Reheating (If Necessary): If your puree has cooled down during the blending process, gently reheat it on the stovetop or in the microwave before serving. Be careful not to overheat, as this can affect the texture and flavor.

Now that you have a solid understanding of basic pureeing techniques, let's explore some tips for preparing delicious pureed meals.

2.3 Tips for Preparing Delicious Pureed Meals

Creating flavorful and satisfying pureed meals requires a combination of technique, creativity, and attention to detail. Here are some tips to help you elevate your pureed cooking game:

Choose Fresh, Seasonal Ingredients: The quality of your ingredients will greatly impact the flavor and texture of your pureed dishes. Opt for fresh, seasonal produce whenever possible, and don't be afraid to experiment with different varieties to add depth and complexity to your recipes.

Wash and Prepare Ingredients: Wash and prepare your chosen ingredients by peeling, chopping, and removing any seeds or pits as needed. For fruits and vegetables, aim for uniform pieces to ensure even cooking and blending.

Cook or Steam Ingredients: Depending on the ingredients you're using, you may need to cook or steam them until they're soft and tender. This helps to enhance their flavor and texture while making them easier to puree.

Blend to Perfection: Once your ingredients are cooked, transfer them to your blender or food processor and blend until smooth and creamy. Use the appropriate speed and blending time to achieve the desired consistency.

Adjust Thickness or Thinness: If your puree is too thick, you can thin it out with a splash of liquid such as water, broth, or milk. Conversely, if it's too thin, you can thicken it with ingredients like cooked rice, potatoes, or beans.

Balance Flavors and Textures: Pureed dishes can sometimes lack complexity, so it's essential to balance flavors and textures to keep things interesting. Incorporate a variety of ingredients, such as herbs, spices, citrus zest, or nuts, to add layers of flavor and crunch.

Incorporate Protein: Adding protein to your pureed meals not only boosts their nutritional value but also helps create a more satisfying and filling dish. Try incorporating lean meats, poultry, fish, tofu, beans, or legumes into your recipes for added protein.

Experiment with Seasonings and Herbs: Don't be afraid to get creative with your seasoning blends and herb combinations. Experiment with different spices, such as cumin, coriander, paprika, or curry powder, to add depth and complexity to your purees. Fresh herbs, such as basil, parsley, cilantro, or mint, can also brighten up the flavor of your dishes.

Add Texture with Garnishes: While pureed dishes are smooth and creamy by nature, adding a variety of garnishes can help add texture and visual appeal. Try topping your purees with crunchy croutons, toasted nuts or seeds, crispy bacon or prosciutto, fresh herbs, or a drizzle of flavorful oil.

Don't Forget About Seasoning: Seasoning is crucial in pureed cooking, as blending can sometimes mute flavors. Taste your puree as you go and adjust the seasoning as needed with salt, pepper, herbs, spices, or acid (such as lemon juice or vinegar) to balance the flavors and enhance the overall taste.

Experiment with Different Cooking Methods: While blending is the primary method of pureeing, don't limit yourself to just one technique. Experiment with different cooking methods, such as roasting, steaming, sautéing, or braising, to develop depth of flavor and complexity in your pureed dishes.

Season to Taste: Taste your puree and season it with salt, pepper, herbs, spices, or other flavorings to enhance its taste. Don't be afraid to experiment with different seasonings to find the perfect balance of flavors.

Get Creative with Presentation: Just because your dish is pureed doesn't mean it has to be boring! Get creative with how you plate and present your purees, using garnishes, sauces, and decorative elements to elevate the visual appeal of your dishes.

By incorporating these tips into your pureed cooking repertoire, you'll be well on your way to creating delicious and satisfying meals that are sure to impress even the most discerning palates.

2.4 Choosing Ingredients for Purees

When it comes to selecting ingredients for purees, the possibilities are endless. Here are some ideas to inspire your culinary creations:

Fruits: Choose ripe and flavorful fruits such as bananas, berries, mangoes, peaches, or apples. These can be enjoyed on their own or combined with other ingredients to create delicious fruit purees.

Vegetables: Opt for a variety of colorful vegetables like carrots, sweet potatoes, spinach, broccoli, or bell peppers. Roasting or steaming vegetables before pureeing can enhance their natural sweetness and flavor.

Grains: Incorporate cooked grains such as rice, quinoa, oats, or barley into your purees for added texture and nutrition. Cooked grains can be blended with fruits or vegetables to create hearty and satisfying meals.

Legumes: Beans, lentils, and chickpeas are excellent sources of protein and fiber. Cooked legumes can be pureed into creamy dips, spreads, or soups for a nutritious and filling meal option.

Meats and Poultry: Cooked meats and poultry can be pureed into smooth and savory purees for added protein. Try blending chicken, turkey, beef, or fish with vegetables and herbs for a flavorful meal.

Dairy and Alternatives: Dairy products like yogurt, milk, or cheese can add creaminess and richness to your purees. For those with lactose intolerance or dairy allergies, alternatives like almond milk, coconut milk, or tofu can be used instead.

2.5 Thickening and Thinning Purees

Achieving the perfect consistency is essential when it comes to purees. Here are some techniques for thickening or thinning your purees to suit your preferences:

Thickening Agents: If your puree is too thin, you can thicken it using various ingredients such as:

- Cooked grains: Add cooked rice, quinoa, or oats to your puree and blend until smooth.
- Starchy vegetables: Potatoes, sweet potatoes, and squash are naturally starchy and can help thicken purees when blended.
- Nut butters: Peanut butter, almond butter, or cashew butter can add thickness and richness to fruit or vegetable purees.
- Dairy products: Greek yogurt, cream cheese, or sour cream can be used to thicken purees while adding creaminess and flavor.

Thinning Agents: If your puree is too thick, you can thin it out using liquids such as:

- Water: Adding water is the simplest way to thin out a puree without altering its flavor.
- Broth or stock: Vegetable, chicken, or beef broth can add flavor while thinning out purees for soups or sauces.
- Milk or milk alternatives: Dairy milk, almond milk, coconut milk, or soy milk can add creaminess and richness while thinning purees.
- Adjusting Consistency: Gradually add thickening or thinning agents to your puree until you achieve the desired consistency. Blend the mixture thoroughly to ensure even distribution of ingredients.

2.6 Flavor Boosters for Purees

Elevate the flavor of your purees with these simple yet impactful flavor boosters:

Herbs and Spices: Fresh or dried herbs and spices can add depth and complexity to your purees. Experiment with combinations like basil and garlic, cilantro and lime, or cinnamon and nutmeg to enhance the taste.

Citrus Zest: Grated citrus zest from lemons, limes, or oranges can add brightness and freshness to fruit purees. Use a microplane grater to zest the fruit directly into your blender or food processor.

Nutritional Yeast: Nutritional yeast is a versatile ingredient that adds a savory, cheesy flavor to purees. Sprinkle it into soups, sauces, or vegetable purees for an extra boost of umami.

Roasted Garlic: Roasting garlic cloves in the oven until golden and caramelized can mellow their flavor and add richness to purees. Blend roasted garlic with vegetables or legumes for a deliciously savory puree.

Infused Oils: Infuse olive oil, coconut oil, or sesame oil with herbs, spices, or aromatics to add depth of flavor to your purees. Drizzle infused oils over finished dishes for a gourmet touch.

2.7 Pureeing Techniques

Mastering the art of pureeing requires a combination of technique and practice. Here are some tips for achieving perfect purees every time:

Start with Small Batches: When pureeing foods, start with small batches to ensure even blending and a smoother consistency. Overcrowding the blender or food processor can result in uneven purees.

Blend in Stages: For larger batches of purees, blend the ingredients in stages to ensure thorough mixing and even texture. Start with the toughest or largest ingredients and gradually add the rest.

Use Liquid Wisely: Adding liquid to your purees helps facilitate blending and achieve the desired consistency. However, it's essential to add liquid gradually to avoid making the puree too thin.

Scrape Down Sides: Periodically stop the blender or food processor and scrape down the sides with a silicone spatula to ensure all ingredients are evenly blended. This helps prevent lumps or chunks from forming.

Adjust Speed and Time: Experiment with different blending speeds and times to achieve the perfect consistency for your purees. Start with a low speed and gradually increase as needed, blending until smooth.

Test for Consistency: Once blended, test the consistency of your puree by spooning a small amount onto a plate. It should be smooth, creamy, and free of lumps or fibrous bits. Adjust thickness or thinness as needed.

2.8 Storing and Reheating Pureed Foods

Proper storage and reheating are essential for maintaining the quality and safety of pureed foods. Here's how to store and reheat your purees:

Refrigeration: Transfer leftover pureed foods to airtight containers and store them in the refrigerator for up to three to four days. Label the containers with the date to track freshness.

Freezing: To extend the shelf life of pureed foods, freeze them in individual portions using ice cube trays or freezer bags. Once frozen, transfer the cubes or portions to a labeled freezer bag for easy storage.

Reheating: When reheating pureed foods, use a microwave, stovetop, or steam oven to gently warm them until heated through. Stir the puree occasionally to ensure even heating and prevent hot spots.

Avoid Repeated Freezing and Thawing: To maintain the quality of pureed foods, avoid repeated freezing and thawing. Instead, portion out the desired amount before freezing to minimize waste.

Check for Signs of Spoilage: Before consuming refrigerated or frozen pureed foods, inspect them for any signs of spoilage, such as off odor, mold growth, or unusual texture. Discard any spoiled or questionable batches.

CHAPTER 3: PUREE-FRIENDLY RECIPES FOR ADULTS

BREAKFAST RECIPES

Difficulty swallowing, medically known as dysphagia, can arise from various causes such as neurological disorders, muscle weakness, or structural abnormalities in the throat or esophagus. This condition can significantly impact one's ability to consume solid foods, leading to nutritional deficiencies and discomfort.

Additionally, adults undergoing oral surgery may experience temporary difficulty in chewing and swallowing due to pain, swelling, or restrictions on their diet during the recovery period. In both cases, it's essential to find alternative ways to meet nutritional needs while ensuring that the food is easy to swallow and gentle on the healing tissues.

Breakfast blends offer a solution to these challenges by providing nourishing options that are soft, smooth, and easy to swallow. By incorporating nutritious ingredients into creamy textures, these blends offer a comforting way to start the day without causing further discomfort or strain on the throat.

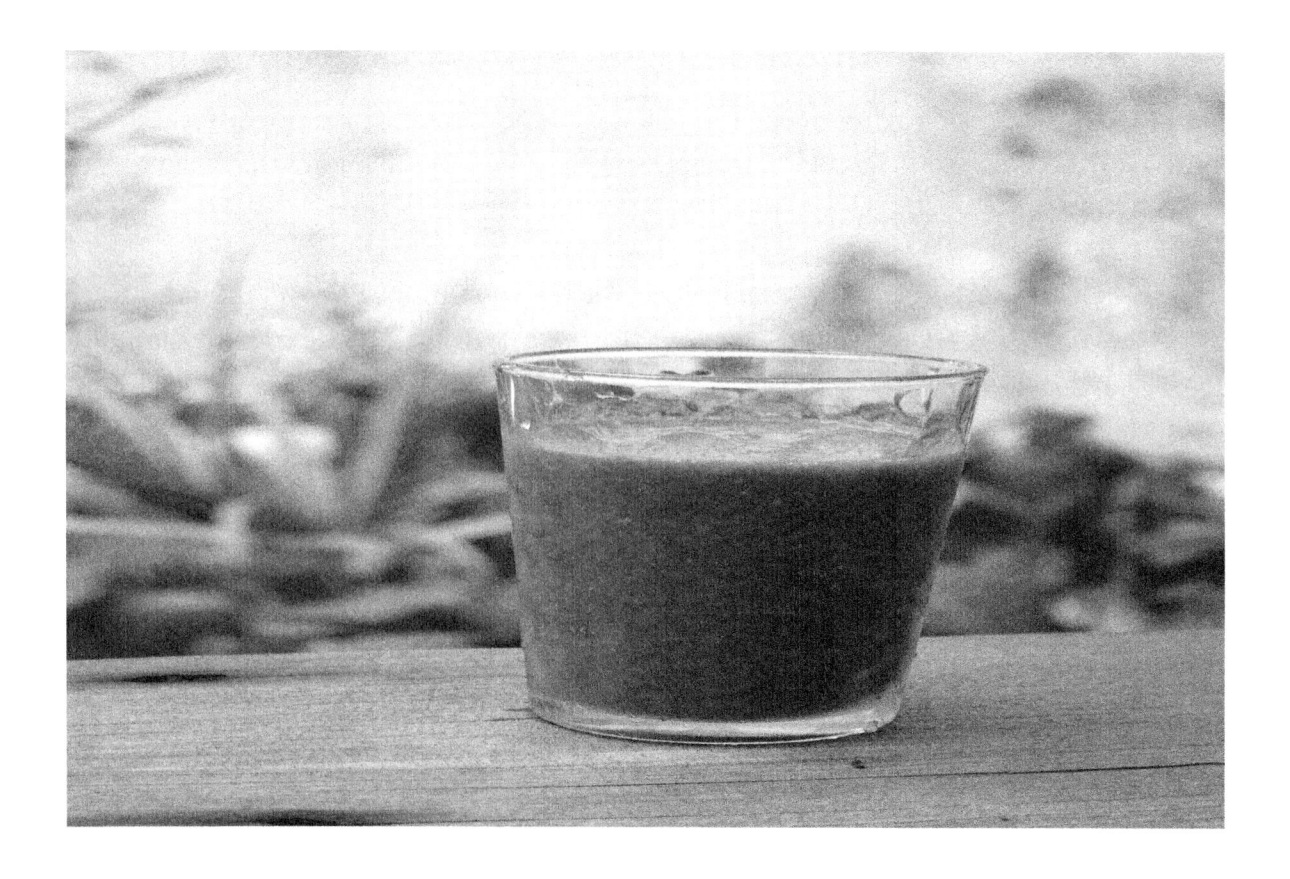

Green Smoothie Puree

Ingredients:
- 1 cup spinach
- 1/2 ripe avocado
- 1/2 cup Greek yogurt
- 1/2 cup almond milk
- 1 scoop vanilla protein powder
- 1 tablespoon honey or maple syrup (optional)

Instructions:
- Combine all ingredients in a blender.

- Blend until smooth and creamy.

- Adjust sweetness with honey or maple syrup if desired.

- Serve chilled.

Nutritional Benefits: This smoothie provides a good source of protein from Greek yogurt and protein powder, healthy fats from avocado, and vitamins and minerals from spinach.

Creamy Berry Oatmeal Puree

Ingredients:
- 1/2 cup rolled oats
- 1 cup milk (dairy or plant-based)
- 1/2 cup mixed berries (such as strawberries, blueberries, raspberries)
- 1 tablespoon chia seeds
- 1 tablespoon almond butter or peanut butter
- 1 tablespoon honey or maple syrup (optional)

Instructions:
- In a saucepan, combine rolled oats and milk.
- Cook over medium heat, stirring occasionally, until oats are soft and creamy.
- Add mixed berries and chia seeds to the saucepan and cook for an additional 2-3 minutes.
- Remove from heat and stir in almond butter and honey or maple syrup if desired.
- Allow to cool slightly, then transfer to a blender.
- Blend until smooth and creamy.
- Serve warm or chilled.

Nutritional Benefits: This puree offers a blend of complex carbohydrates from oats, antioxidants from mixed berries, omega-3 fatty acids from chia seeds, and protein and healthy fats from almond butter.

Vegetable Breakfast Puree

Ingredients:
- 1/2 cup cooked quinoa
- 1/2 cup steamed spinach
- 1/2 cup steamed carrots
- 1/4 cup cooked lentils
- 1 tablespoon olive oil
- 1 teaspoon lemon juice
- Salt and pepper to taste

Instructions:
- In a blender, combine cooked quinoa, steamed spinach, steamed carrots, cooked lentils, olive oil, lemon juice, salt, and pepper.

- Blend until smooth and creamy, adding water or vegetable broth as needed to reach desired consistency.

- Transfer puree to a saucepan and heat gently over low heat until warmed through.

- Serve warm.

Nutritional Benefits: This puree is rich in fiber from quinoa and lentils, vitamins and minerals from spinach and carrots, and heart-healthy fats from olive oil.

Creamy Banana Nut Breakfast Puree

Ingredients:
- 1 ripe banana
- 1/4 cup Greek yogurt
- 2 tablespoons almond butter or peanut butter
- 1/4 teaspoon ground cinnamon
- 1 tablespoon honey or maple syrup (optional)
- 1/4 cup milk (dairy or plant-based)

Instructions:
- In a blender, combine ripe banana, Greek yogurt, almond butter or peanut butter, ground cinnamon, honey or maple syrup, and milk.

- Blend until smooth and creamy.

- Adjust sweetness with honey or maple syrup if desired.

- Serve chilled.

Nutritional Benefits: This puree provides a good source of potassium from banana, protein from Greek yogurt and nut butter, and healthy fats from almond butter or peanut butter.

Pumpkin Spice Breakfast Puree

Ingredients:
- 1/2 cup canned pumpkin puree
- 1/2 cup Greek yogurt
- 1/4 cup rolled oats
- 1 tablespoon honey or maple syrup
- 1/4 teaspoon ground cinnamon
- 1/8 teaspoon ground nutmeg
- 1/8 teaspoon ground ginger
- 1/8 teaspoon ground cloves
- 1/4 cup milk (dairy or plant-based)

Instructions:
- In a blender, combine pumpkin puree, Greek yogurt, rolled oats, honey or maple syrup, ground cinnamon, ground nutmeg, ground ginger, ground cloves, and milk.

- Blend until smooth and creamy.

- Adjust sweetness with honey or maple syrup if desired.

- Serve chilled or warmed.

Nutritional Benefits: This puree is high in fiber from pumpkin and oats, protein from Greek yogurt, and essential vitamins and minerals from spices like cinnamon, nutmeg, ginger, and cloves.

Creamy Coconut Mango Chia Pudding Puree

Ingredients:
- 1 ripe mango, peeled and diced
- 1/2 cup coconut milk
- 2 tablespoons chia seeds
- 1 tablespoon honey or maple syrup
- 1/2 teaspoon vanilla extract

Instructions:
- In a blender, combine ripe mango, coconut milk, chia seeds, honey or maple syrup, and vanilla extract.
- Blend until smooth and creamy.
- Transfer mixture to a bowl or jar and refrigerate for at least 4 hours, or overnight, until thickened.
- Serve chilled.

Nutritional Benefits: This puree is rich in fiber from chia seeds, vitamins and minerals from mango, and healthy fats from coconut milk.

Creamy Spinach and Feta Breakfast Puree

Ingredients:
- 1 cup cooked quinoa
- 1 cup cooked spinach, drained
- 1/4 cup crumbled feta cheese
- 2 tablespoons Greek yogurt
- 1 tablespoon olive oil
- 1 teaspoon lemon juice
- Salt and pepper to taste

Instructions:

- In a blender, combine cooked quinoa, cooked spinach, crumbled feta cheese, Greek yogurt, olive oil, lemon juice, salt, and pepper.

- Blend until smooth and creamy, adding water or vegetable broth as needed to reach desired consistency.

- Transfer puree to a saucepan and heat gently over low heat until warmed through.

- Serve warm.

Nutritional Benefits: This puree is a good source of protein from quinoa and Greek yogurt, iron and calcium from spinach, and flavor from feta cheese.

Soft Blueberry Pancakes with Yogurt Sauce

Ingredients:
- 1/2 cup rolled oats
- 1 ripe banana
- 2 eggs
- 1/4 cup Greek yogurt
- 1/2 cup fresh or frozen blueberries
- 1 tablespoon honey or maple syrup
- 1/2 teaspoon vanilla extract
- Butter or oil for cooking

Instructions:
- In a blender, combine rolled oats, ripe banana, eggs, Greek yogurt, honey or maple syrup, and vanilla extract.

- Blend until smooth and creamy.

- Heat a non-stick skillet over medium heat and lightly grease with butter or oil.

- Pour small amounts of batter onto the skillet to form pancakes.

- Drop blueberries onto each pancake.

- Cook until bubbles form on the surface of the pancakes, then flip and cook until golden brown on the other side.

- Serve warm with a dollop of Greek yogurt on top.

Nutritional Benefits: These pancakes offer a blend of complex carbohydrates from oats and banana, protein from eggs and Greek yogurt, and antioxidants from blueberries.

Soft Breakfast Casserole with Sweet Potatoes and Turkey

Ingredients:
- 2 cups cooked sweet potatoes, mashed
- 1 cup cooked ground turkey
- 1/2 cup cooked spinach, drained
- 1/4 cup shredded cheddar cheese
- 4 eggs
- 1/4 cup milk or cream
- Salt and pepper to taste

Instructions:
- Preheat the oven to 350°F (175°C). Grease a baking dish with butter or cooking spray.

- In a bowl, combine mashed sweet potatoes, cooked ground turkey, cooked spinach, and shredded cheddar cheese.

- Spread the mixture evenly in the prepared baking dish.

- In another bowl, whisk together eggs, milk or cream, salt, and pepper.

- Pour the egg mixture over the sweet potato mixture in the baking dish.

- Bake for 25-30 minutes, or until the eggs are set and the top is lightly golden.

- Allow to cool slightly, then cut into squares and serve warm.

Nutritional Benefits: This breakfast casserole provides a balance of protein from ground turkey and eggs, vitamins and minerals from sweet potatoes and spinach, and calcium from cheddar cheese.

Creamy Pumpkin Breakfast Smoothie

Ingredients:
- 1/2 cup canned pumpkin puree
- 1/2 ripe banana
- 1/2 cup Greek yogurt
- 1/4 cup rolled oats
- 1 tablespoon almond butter or peanut butter
- 1 tablespoon honey or maple syrup
- 1/2 teaspoon ground cinnamon
- 1/4 teaspoon ground nutmeg
- 1/4 teaspoon ground ginger
- 1/4 teaspoon vanilla extract
- 1 cup milk or any preferred milk alternative

Instructions:
- In a blender, combine pumpkin puree, ripe banana, Greek yogurt, rolled oats, almond butter or peanut butter, honey or maple syrup, ground cinnamon, ground nutmeg, ground ginger, vanilla extract, and milk.

- Blend until smooth and creamy.

- Adjust sweetness with honey or maple syrup if desired.

- Serve chilled.

Nutritional Benefits: This smoothie is high in fiber from pumpkin and oats, protein from Greek yogurt, and essential vitamins and minerals from spices like cinnamon, nutmeg, and ginger.

Soft Baked Apples with Yogurt and Granola

Ingredients:
- 2 apples, cored and sliced
- 2 tablespoons unsalted butter, melted
- 2 tablespoons brown sugar
- 1/2 teaspoon ground cinnamon
- 1 cup Greek yogurt or plant-based yogurt
- 1/2 cup granola

Instructions:
- Preheat the oven to 350°F (175°C).

- In a bowl, toss the sliced apples with melted butter, brown sugar, and ground cinnamon until evenly coated.

- Arrange the apple slices in a single layer in a baking dish.

- Bake for 20-25 minutes, or until the apples are soft and tender.

- Serve the baked apples warm, topped with Greek yogurt and granola.

Soft Scrambled Tofu with Spinach and Cheese

Ingredients:

- 1 block (14 oz) firm tofu, drained and crumbled
- 1 tablespoon olive oil
- 1 cup fresh spinach leaves
- 1/4 cup shredded cheese (such as cheddar or mozzarella)
- Salt and pepper to taste

Instructions:

- Heat the olive oil in a non-stick skillet over medium heat.

- Add the crumbled tofu to the skillet and cook for 3-4 minutes, stirring occasionally.

- Add the fresh spinach leaves to the skillet and cook until wilted.

- Sprinkle shredded cheese over the tofu and spinach mixture.

- Continue cooking until the cheese is melted and the tofu is heated through.

- Season with salt and pepper to taste.

- Serve the soft scrambled tofu warm.

Banana Peanut Butter Smoothie

Ingredients:
- 1 ripe banana
- 2 tablespoons peanut butter
- 1 cup milk or any preferred milk alternative
- 1/2 cup Greek yogurt or plant-based yogurt
- 1 tablespoon honey or maple syrup (optional)
- Ice cubes (optional)

Instructions:
- In a blender, combine the ripe banana, peanut butter, milk, Greek yogurt, and honey or maple syrup (if using).

- Add ice cubes if a colder consistency is desired.

- Blend on high speed until smooth and creamy.

- Pour the smoothie into glasses and serve immediately.

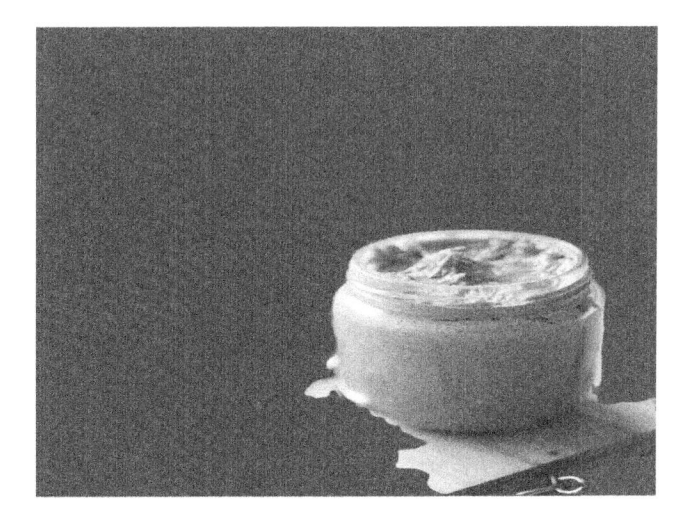

Soft French Toast with Berries and Honey

Ingredients:

- 4 slices of soft bread (such as brioche or challah)
- 2 eggs
- 1/4 cup milk or cream
- 1 teaspoon vanilla extract
- Butter for greasing the skillet
- Mixed berries (such as strawberries, blueberries, raspberries)
- Honey for drizzling

Instructions:

- In a shallow dish, whisk together the eggs, milk, and vanilla extract.
- Dip each slice of bread into the egg mixture, ensuring it is evenly coated.
- Heat a non-stick skillet or griddle over medium heat and grease with butter.
- Cook the soaked bread slices for 2-3 minutes on each side, until golden brown and cooked through.
- Serve the French toast warm, topped with mixed berries and a drizzle of honey.

Creamy Mango Banana Smoothie Bowl

Ingredients:

- 1 ripe banana
- 1/2 cup frozen mango chunks
- 1/2 cup Greek yogurt or plant-based yogurt
- 1/4 cup rolled oats
- 1 tablespoon honey or maple syrup (optional)
- 1/4 cup almond milk or any preferred milk alternative
- Toppings: sliced mango, shredded coconut, chia seeds

Instructions:

- In a blender, combine the ripe banana, frozen mango chunks, Greek yogurt, rolled oats, honey or maple syrup (if using), and almond milk.

- Blend on high speed until smooth and creamy.

- Pour the smoothie into a bowl.

- Arrange sliced mango on top of the smoothie.

- Sprinkle shredded coconut and chia seeds over the smoothie.

- Serve immediately with a spoon.

Soft Boiled Eggs with Toast Soldiers

Ingredients:

- 2 eggs
- 2 slices of soft bread, toasted and cut into strips
- Salt and pepper to taste

Instructions:

- Bring a pot of water to a boil.
- Carefully lower the eggs into the boiling water using a spoon.
- Boil the eggs for 4-5 minutes for a soft yolk.
- Remove the eggs from the water and transfer them to egg cups.
- Gently tap the tops of the eggs with a spoon to crack them open.
- Serve the soft boiled eggs with toast soldiers for dipping.
- Season with salt and pepper to taste.

Creamy Blueberry Banana Smoothie

Ingredients:

- 1 ripe banana
- 1/2 cup frozen blueberries
- 1/2 cup Greek yogurt or plant-based yogurt
- 1/4 cup rolled oats
- 1 tablespoon honey or maple syrup (optional)
- 1/4 cup almond milk or any preferred milk alternative

Instructions:

- In a blender, combine the ripe banana, frozen blueberries, Greek yogurt, rolled oats, honey or maple syrup (if using), and almond milk.

- Blend on high speed until smooth and creamy.

- Pour the smoothie into glasses and serve immediately.

Soft Baked Oatmeal with Berries

Ingredients:

- 1 cup rolled oats
- 1 ripe banana, mashed
- 1 cup milk or any preferred milk alternative
- 1 tablespoon honey or maple syrup
- 1/2 teaspoon ground cinnamon
- 1/2 cup mixed berries (such as strawberries, blueberries, raspberries)
- Optional toppings: Greek yogurt, sliced bananas, chopped nuts

Instructions:

- Preheat the oven to 350°F (175°C). Grease a baking dish with butter or cooking spray.

- In a bowl, combine the rolled oats, mashed banana, milk, honey or maple syrup, and ground cinnamon.

- Gently fold in the mixed berries.

- Pour the oatmeal mixture into the prepared baking dish.

- Bake for 25-30 minutes, or until the oatmeal is set and lightly golden on top.

- Serve the baked oatmeal warm, topped with Greek yogurt, sliced bananas, and chopped nuts if desired.

Soft Ricotta Pancakes with Berry Compote

Ingredients:

- 1 cup all-purpose flour
- 1 tablespoon sugar
- 1 teaspoon baking powder
- 1/4 teaspoon salt
- 1 cup ricotta cheese
- 2 eggs
- 1/2 cup milk or any preferred milk alternative
- 1 teaspoon vanilla extract
- Butter or oil for greasing the skillet
- Berry compote (made by simmering mixed berries with sugar and water)

Instructions:

- In a bowl, whisk together the all-purpose flour, sugar, baking powder, and salt.

- In another bowl, whisk together the ricotta cheese, eggs, milk, and vanilla extract until smooth.

- Gradually add the dry ingredients to the wet ingredients, stirring until just combined.

- Heat a non-stick skillet or griddle over medium heat and lightly grease with butter or oil.

- Pour a small amount of batter onto the skillet to form pancakes.

- Cook until bubbles form on the surface of the pancakes, then flip and cook until golden brown on the other side.

- Serve the ricotta pancakes warm, topped with berry compote.

Burrito with Scrambled Eggs and Avocado

Ingredients:

- 2 large eggs
- 2 tablespoons milk or cream
- Salt and pepper to taste
- 2 large soft tortillas
- 1 ripe avocado, sliced
- Salsa or hot sauce (optional)

Instructions:

- In a bowl, whisk together the eggs, milk or cream, salt, and pepper.
- Heat a non-stick skillet over medium heat.
- Pour the egg mixture into the skillet and scramble until cooked through.
- Warm the soft tortillas in the skillet or microwave.
- Divide the scrambled eggs between the tortillas.
- Top with sliced avocado and salsa or hot sauce if desired.
- Roll up the tortillas to form burritos.
- Serve the breakfast burritos warm.

Creamy Banana Oatmeal

Ingredients:

- 1 ripe banana
- 1/2 cup rolled oats
- 1 cup milk (dairy or plant-based)
- 1/2 teaspoon cinnamon
- 1 tablespoon honey or maple syrup (optional)
- Toppings: sliced bananas, chopped nuts, drizzle of honey (optional)

Instructions:

- In a saucepan, mash the ripe banana until smooth.

- Add the rolled oats, milk, and cinnamon to the saucepan and stir to combine.

- Place the saucepan over medium heat and bring the mixture to a gentle simmer.

- Cook for 5-7 minutes, stirring occasionally, until the oats are soft and creamy.

- If desired, sweeten with honey or maple syrup to taste.

- Serve the oatmeal warm, topped with sliced bananas, chopped nuts, and a drizzle of honey, if desired.

Silken Smoothie

Ingredients:
- 1 ripe avocado
- 1 cup spinach leaves
- 1/2 cup frozen berries (such as strawberries, blueberries, or raspberries)
- 1/2 cup Greek yogurt or plant-based yogurt
- 1 tablespoon honey or maple syrup (optional)
- 1/2 cup water or coconut water

Instructions:
- Cut the avocado in half, remove the pit, and scoop the flesh into a blender.

- Add the spinach leaves, frozen berries, Greek yogurt, honey or maple syrup (if using), and water to the blender.

- Blend on high speed until smooth and creamy.

- If the smoothie is too thick, add more water until desired consistency is reached.

- Taste and adjust sweetness if necessary by adding more honey or maple syrup.

- Pour the smoothie into glasses and serve immediately.

Green Smoothie Bowl

Ingredients:

- 1 ripe banana
- 1/2 cup frozen mango chunks
- 1 cup fresh spinach leaves
- 1/2 cup Greek yogurt or plant-based yogurt
- 1 tablespoon honey or maple syrup (optional)
- 1/4 cup almond milk or any preferred milk alternative
- Toppings: sliced kiwi, shredded coconut, chia seeds

Instructions:

- In a blender, combine the ripe banana, frozen mango chunks, fresh spinach leaves, Greek yogurt, honey or maple syrup (if using), and almond milk.

- Blend on high speed until smooth and creamy.

- Pour the smoothie into a bowl.

- Arrange sliced kiwi on top of the smoothie.

- Sprinkle shredded coconut and chia seeds over the smoothie.

- Serve immediately with a spoon.

Soft Scrambled Eggs with Herbs

Ingredients:

- 2 eggs
- 2 tablespoons milk or cream
- 1 tablespoon unsalted butter or olive oil
- Salt and pepper to taste
- Chopped fresh herbs (such as chives, parsley, or dill)

Instructions:

- In a bowl, whisk together the eggs and milk until well combined.
- Heat the unsalted butter or olive oil in a non-stick skillet over medium heat.
- Pour the egg mixture into the skillet.
- Gently scramble the eggs with a spatula, stirring continuously until they are softly set.
- Season with salt and pepper to taste.
- Sprinkle chopped fresh herbs over the scrambled eggs.
- Serve immediately while warm.

Banana Yogurt Pancakes

Ingredients:
- 1 ripe banana, mashed
- 1/2 cup Greek yogurt or plant-based yogurt
- 1 egg
- 1/2 teaspoon vanilla extract
- 1/2 cup all-purpose flour or oat flour
- 1 teaspoon baking powder
- Pinch of salt
- Butter or oil for greasing the skillet
- Toppings: sliced bananas, Greek yogurt, honey or maple syrup

Instructions:

- In a bowl, combine the mashed banana, Greek yogurt, egg, and vanilla extract.

- In a separate bowl, whisk together the flour, baking powder, and salt.

- Gradually add the dry ingredients to the wet ingredients, stirring until just combined.

- Heat a non-stick skillet or griddle over medium heat and lightly grease with butter or oil.

- Pour a small amount of batter onto the skillet to form pancakes.

- Cook until bubbles form on the surface of the pancakes, then flip and cook until golden brown on the other side.

- Repeat with the remaining batter.

- Serve the pancakes warm, topped with sliced bananas, Greek yogurt, and honey or maple syrup.

HEALING SOUPS AND BROTHS RECIPES

One of the primary benefits of consuming soups and broths lies in their hydrating properties. Both water and electrolytes are essential for maintaining proper bodily functions, and soups, especially those with a high liquid content, serve as an effective means of replenishing fluids. Adequate hydration supports cellular hydration, aids in toxin removal, and promotes overall well-being.

For adults experiencing difficulty swallowing, soups and broths offer a palatable alternative to solid foods. Their smooth consistency and lack of solid particles reduce the risk of choking or aspiration, making them ideal for those with dysphagia or recovering from throat surgery. By facilitating safe and comfortable swallowing, these liquid-based preparations ensure that individuals receive vital nutrients without added strain.

Certain health conditions, such as gastritis, acid reflux, or postoperative gastrointestinal sensitivity, require dietary choices that are gentle on the stomach. Unlike heavy or spicy meals that may exacerbate digestive discomfort, soups and broths provide a soothing option that is easy to digest. Their mild flavors and absence of irritants make them well-tolerated even by individuals with sensitive stomachs, promoting healing and comfort.

Despite their seemingly simple composition, healing soups and broths are nutritional powerhouses packed with essential vitamins, minerals, and macronutrients necessary for optimal health. Depending on the ingredients used, these liquid concoctions can deliver a diverse array of nutrients that support bodily functions and promote overall wellness.

Vegetable-based soups, for example, are rich in vitamins A, C, and K, as well as folate, potassium, and fiber, all of which play crucial roles in immune function, wound healing, and cardiovascular health. Similarly, bone broths derived from animal sources are prized for their high protein content, collagen, gelatin, and amino acids such as glycine and proline, which support joint health, gut integrity, and skin elasticity.

By incorporating a variety of nutrient-dense ingredients, healing soups and broths offer a convenient and efficient means of meeting daily nutritional requirements without the need for complex meal planning or supplementation. Their versatility allows for endless customization based on individual preferences and dietary needs, ensuring that everyone can reap the benefits of these nourishing elixirs.

Creamy Carrot Ginger Soup

Ingredients:
- 1 lb carrots, peeled and chopped
- 1 small onion, chopped
- 2 cloves garlic, minced
- 1-inch piece of fresh ginger, peeled and minced
- 4 cups vegetable broth
- 1 cup coconut milk
- Salt and pepper to taste

Instructions:
- In a large pot, sauté the onion, garlic, and ginger until fragrant.

- Add the chopped carrots and vegetable broth to the pot. Bring to a boil, then reduce heat and simmer until the carrots are tender.

- Using an immersion blender or countertop blender, puree the soup until smooth.

- Stir in the coconut milk and season with salt and pepper to taste.

- Simmer for an additional 5 minutes, then serve hot.

Spinach and Avocado Soup:

Ingredients:
- 6 cups fresh spinach
- 1 ripe avocado, peeled and pitted
- 2 cups vegetable broth
- 1 clove garlic, minced
- Juice of 1 lemon
- Salt and pepper to taste

Instructions:
- In a blender, combine the spinach, avocado, vegetable broth, garlic, and lemon juice.
- Blend until smooth, adding more broth if needed to reach desired consistency.
- Season with salt and pepper to taste.
- Transfer the soup to a pot and heat gently over medium-low heat until warmed through.
- Serve hot, garnished with a slice of lemon if desired.

Broccoli and Cauliflower Puree

Ingredients:
- 1 head broccoli, chopped
- 1 head cauliflower, chopped
- 1 onion, chopped
- 2 cloves garlic, minced
- 4 cups vegetable broth
- 1 cup coconut milk
- Salt and pepper to taste

Instructions:
- In a large pot, sauté the onion and garlic until softened.

- Add the chopped broccoli, cauliflower, and vegetable broth to the pot. Bring to a boil, then reduce heat and simmer until the vegetables are tender.

- Using an immersion blender or countertop blender, puree the soup until smooth.

- Stir in the coconut milk and season with salt and pepper to taste.

- Simmer for an additional 5 minutes, then serve hot.

Creamy Mushroom Soup

Ingredients:
- 1 lb mushrooms, sliced (any variety)
- 1 onion, chopped
- 2 cloves garlic, minced
- 4 cups vegetable broth
- 1 cup coconut milk
- 2 tbsp olive oil
- Salt and pepper to taste

Instructions:
- In a large pot, heat the olive oil over medium heat. Add the onion and garlic, and sauté until softened.

- Add the sliced mushrooms to the pot and cook until they release their juices and become tender.

- Pour in the vegetable broth and bring to a simmer. Let it cook for about 10 minutes.

- Using an immersion blender or countertop blender, puree the soup until smooth.

- Stir in the coconut milk and season with salt and pepper to taste.

- Simmer for an additional 5 minutes before serving hot.

Sweet Potato and Coconut Soup

Ingredients:
- 2 large sweet potatoes, peeled and diced
- 1 onion, chopped
- 2 cloves garlic, minced
- 1 can (14 oz) coconut milk
- 4 cups vegetable broth
- 2 tbsp olive oil
- Salt and pepper to taste

Instructions:
- In a large pot, heat the olive oil over medium heat. Add the onion and garlic, and sauté until softened.

- Add the diced sweet potatoes and vegetable broth to the pot. Bring to a boil, then reduce heat and simmer until the sweet potatoes are tender.

- Using an immersion blender or countertop blender, puree the soup until smooth.

- Stir in the coconut milk and season with salt and pepper to taste.

- Simmer for an additional 5 minutes before serving hot.

Pea and Mint Puree

Ingredients:
- 2 cups frozen peas
- 1 onion, chopped
- 2 cloves garlic, minced
- 4 cups vegetable broth
- 1/4 cup fresh mint leaves
- 2 tbsp olive oil
- Salt and pepper to taste

Instructions:
- In a large pot, heat the olive oil over medium heat. Add the onion and garlic, and sauté until softened.
- Add the frozen peas and vegetable broth to the pot. Bring to a boil, then reduce heat and simmer for about 5-7 minutes until the peas are tender.
- Remove the pot from heat and stir in the fresh mint leaves.
- Using an immersion blender or countertop blender, puree the soup until smooth.
- Season with salt and pepper to taste.
- Serve hot, optionally garnished with a sprig of fresh mint.

Creamy Asparagus Soup

Ingredients:
- 1 lb asparagus, trimmed and chopped
- 1 onion, chopped
- 2 cloves garlic, minced
- 4 cups vegetable broth
- 1/2 cup coconut milk
- 2 tbsp olive oil
- Salt and pepper to taste

Instructions:
- In a large pot, heat the olive oil over medium heat. Add the onion and garlic, and sauté until softened.

- Add the chopped asparagus and vegetable broth to the pot. Bring to a boil, then reduce heat and simmer until the asparagus is tender.

- Using an immersion blender or countertop blender, puree the soup until smooth.

- Stir in the coconut milk and season with salt and pepper to taste.

- Simmer for an additional 5 minutes before serving hot.

Tomato and Red Pepper Bisque

Ingredients:
- 4 large tomatoes, chopped
- 2 red bell peppers, chopped
- 1 onion, chopped
- 2 cloves garlic, minced
- 4 cups vegetable broth
- 1/4 cup tomato paste
- 2 tbsp olive oil
- Salt and pepper to taste

Instructions:
- In a large pot, heat the olive oil over medium heat. Add the onion and garlic, and sauté until softened.

- Add the chopped tomatoes, red bell peppers, vegetable broth, and tomato paste to the pot. Bring to a boil, then reduce heat and simmer until the vegetables are tender.

- Using an immersion blender or countertop blender, puree the soup until smooth.

- Season with salt and pepper to taste.

- Serve hot, optionally garnished with fresh basil or a drizzle of olive oil.

Lentil and Coconut Curry Soup

Ingredients:
- 1 cup dried red lentils
- 1 onion, chopped
- 2 cloves garlic, minced
- 1-inch piece of ginger, peeled and minced
- 1 can (14 oz) coconut milk
- 4 cups vegetable broth
- 2 tbsp curry powder
- 2 tbsp olive oil
- Salt and pepper to taste

Instructions:
- In a large pot, heat the olive oil over medium heat. Add the onion, garlic, and ginger, and sauté until softened.

- Add the curry powder to the pot and cook for another minute until fragrant.

- Rinse the red lentils under cold water, then add them to the pot along with the vegetable broth and coconut milk.

- Bring the soup to a boil, then reduce heat and simmer for about 20-25 minutes, or until the lentils are tender.

- Using an immersion blender or countertop blender, puree the soup until smooth.

- Season with salt and pepper to taste.

- Serve hot, optionally garnished with chopped cilantro or a squeeze of lime juice.

Creamy Cauliflower and Leek Soup

Ingredients:
- 1 head cauliflower, chopped
- 2 leeks, white and light green parts only, chopped
- 2 cloves garlic, minced
- 4 cups vegetable broth
- 1/2 cup coconut milk
- 2 tbsp olive oil
- Salt and pepper to taste

Instructions:
- In a large pot, heat the olive oil over medium heat. Add the leeks and garlic, and sauté until softened.

- Add the chopped cauliflower and vegetable broth to the pot. Bring to a boil, then reduce heat and simmer until the cauliflower is tender.

- Using an immersion blender or countertop blender, puree the soup until smooth.

- Stir in the coconut milk and season with salt and pepper to taste.

- Simmer for an additional 5 minutes before serving hot.

Smooth and Creamy Mashed Potatoes

Ingredients:
- 4 medium potatoes, peeled and diced
- 1/4 cup milk (or dairy-free alternative)
- 2 tablespoons unsalted butter (or olive oil for a dairy-free option)
- Salt and pepper to taste

Instructions:
- Boil potatoes in salted water until tender. Drain.
- Mash potatoes with milk and butter until smooth.
- Season with salt and pepper to taste.
- Serve hot.

Garlic Infused Cauliflower Mash

Ingredients:
- 1 head cauliflower, chopped into florets
- 2 cloves garlic, minced
- 2 tablespoons olive oil
- Salt and pepper to taste

Instructions:
- Steam or boil cauliflower until very tender.

- In a pan, sauté minced garlic in olive oil until fragrant.

- Mash cauliflower and garlic together until smooth.

- Season with salt and pepper to taste.

- Serve as a healthy alternative to mashed potatoes.

Creamed Spinach with Nutmeg

Ingredients:
- 1 lb fresh spinach, washed and trimmed
- 1/2 cup milk (or dairy-free alternative)
- 2 tablespoons unsalted butter (or olive oil)
- 1/4 teaspoon ground nutmeg
- Salt and pepper to taste

Instructions:
- Blanch spinach in boiling water for 1-2 minutes, then drain and squeeze out excess water.

- In a saucepan, melt butter over medium heat. Add blanched spinach and cook until wilted.

- Stir in milk and nutmeg, then simmer for 5 minutes.

- Puree the mixture until smooth using a blender or immersion blender.

- Season with salt and pepper to taste.

- Serve warm as a nutritious side dish.

Pureed Carrots with Ginger

Ingredients:
- 1 lb carrots, peeled and chopped
- 1 tablespoon fresh ginger, grated
- 2 cups vegetable broth
- 2 tablespoons olive oil
- Salt and pepper to taste

Instructions:
- In a pot, heat olive oil over medium heat. Add grated ginger and sauté for 1 minute.

- Add chopped carrots and vegetable broth to the pot. Bring to a boil, then reduce heat and simmer until carrots are tender.

- Allow the mixture to cool slightly, then puree until smooth using a blender or immersion blender.

- Season with salt and pepper to taste.

- Serve as a flavorful and nutritious side dish.

Velvety Pumpkin Puree

Ingredients:
- 1 small pumpkin, peeled, seeded, and diced
- 1 onion, chopped
- 2 cloves garlic, minced
- 2 cups vegetable broth
- 1/2 teaspoon ground cinnamon
- Salt and pepper to taste

Instructions:
- In a large pot, sauté chopped onion and minced garlic until softened.

- Add diced pumpkin and vegetable broth to the pot. Bring to a boil, then reduce heat and simmer until pumpkin is tender.

- Allow the mixture to cool slightly, then puree until smooth using a blender or immersion blender.

- Stir in ground cinnamon, then season with salt and pepper to taste.

- Serve warm as a comforting and nutritious puree.

Beetroot and Potato Mash

Ingredients:
- 2 medium beetroots, peeled and diced
- 2 medium potatoes, peeled and diced
- 1/4 cup milk (or dairy-free alternative)
- 2 tablespoons unsalted butter (or olive oil)
- Salt and pepper to taste

Instructions:
- Boil diced beetroots and potatoes in salted water until tender, drain.
- Mash beetroots and potatoes together with milk and butter until smooth.
- Season with salt and pepper to taste.
- Serve as a vibrant and nutritious side dish.

Zucchini and Basil Puree

Ingredients:
- 2 medium zucchinis, chopped
- 1/4 cup fresh basil leaves
- 2 tablespoons olive oil
- 1 tablespoon lemon juice
- Salt and pepper to taste

Instructions:
- Steam or boil chopped zucchinis until very tender.

- In a blender, combine cooked zucchinis, fresh basil leaves, olive oil, and lemon juice.

- Puree until smooth, adding water as needed to reach desired consistency.

- Season with salt and pepper to taste.

- Serve chilled as a refreshing and nutritious puree.

Broccoli and Cheese Puree

Ingredients:
- 2 cups broccoli florets
- 1/2 cup cheddar cheese, shredded
- 1/4 cup milk (or dairy-free alternative)
- 1 tablespoon unsalted butter (or olive oil)
- Salt and pepper to taste

Instructions:
- Steam or boil broccoli florets until very tender.

- In a saucepan, melt butter over medium heat. Add cooked broccoli, shredded cheddar cheese, and milk.

- Cook until cheese is melted and mixture is heated through.

- Puree the mixture until smooth using a blender or immersion blender.

- Season with salt and pepper to taste.

- Serve warm as a comforting and nutritious puree.

Sweet Potato and Coconut Puree

Ingredients:
- 2 medium sweet potatoes, peeled and diced
- 1/2 cup coconut milk
- 2 tablespoons unsalted butter (or coconut oil)
- 1 tablespoon maple syrup (optional)
- Salt to taste

Instructions:
- Boil diced sweet potatoes in salted water until tender. Drain.
- In a saucepan, combine cooked sweet potatoes, coconut milk, and butter.
- Cook over medium heat until heated through.
- Puree the mixture until smooth using a blender or immersion blender.
- Stir in maple syrup if desired, then season with salt to taste.
- Serve as a deliciously sweet and nutritious puree.

Creamy Asparagus and Potato Puree

Ingredients:
- 1 bunch asparagus, trimmed and chopped
- 2 medium potatoes, peeled and diced
- 2 cups vegetable broth
- 1/4 cup heavy cream (or coconut cream for a dairy-free option)
- 2 tablespoons unsalted butter (or olive oil)
- Salt and pepper to taste

Instructions:
- In a pot, combine chopped asparagus, diced potatoes, and vegetable broth. Bring to a boil, then reduce heat and simmer until vegetables are tender.

- Allow the mixture to cool slightly, then puree until smooth using a blender or immersion blender.

- Stir in heavy cream and butter until well combined.

- Season with salt and pepper to taste.

- Serve hot as a luxurious and nutritious puree.

DESSERT RECIPES

Some of the dessert ingredients are;

Avocado is a nutrient-rich fruit packed with heart-healthy fats, fiber, and various vitamins and minerals. In this recipe, avocado serves as a creamy base, offering a satisfying texture without spiking blood sugar levels.

Nutritional Values: Avocados are low in carbohydrates and naturally sugar-free, making them an excellent choice for managing diabetes. The addition of cocoa powder provides antioxidants and a rich chocolate flavor without added sugars.
Scientific Benefits: Avocados may help regulate blood sugar levels and promote cardiovascular health due to their monounsaturated fat content. Cocoa has been linked to improved mood and relaxation due to its flavonoid content.

Bananas are a good source of potassium, which supports heart health and may help lower blood pressure. Chia seeds add fiber, omega-3 fatty acids, and protein, contributing to a satisfying and nutritious dessert option.
Nutritional Values: Bananas are naturally sweet but have a relatively low glycemic index, making them suitable for diabetic individuals when consumed in moderation. Chia seeds provide a gel-like texture when mixed with liquid, aiding in swallowing for those with oral surgery or swallowing difficulties.
Scientific Benefits: The fiber in bananas and chia seeds can help stabilize blood sugar levels and promote digestive health. Omega-3 fatty acids from chia seeds may have anti-inflammatory effects, benefiting overall health.

Mangoes are rich in vitamins A and C, as well as antioxidants, which support immune function and skin health. Coconut milk adds creaminess and flavor while being dairy-free and lower in sugar than traditional ice cream.
Nutritional Values: Mangoes are relatively low in calories and have a moderate glycemic index, making them suitable for diabetes management when portion-controlled. Coconut milk provides healthy fats and can be a satisfying alternative to dairy-based desserts.
Scientific Benefits: The vitamins and antioxidants in mangoes may help reduce inflammation and oxidative stress in the body. Coconut milk contains medium-chain triglycerides (MCTs), which are easily digestible and may provide quick energy.

Cinnamon-Spiced Sweet Potato Mash

Ingredients:
- 2 medium sweet potatoes, peeled and cubed
- 1 teaspoon ground cinnamon
- 1 tablespoon coconut oil
- Pinch of salt

Instructions:
- Boil or steam the sweet potato cubes until tender.
- Drain and transfer to a mixing bowl.
- Add ground cinnamon, coconut oil, and a pinch of salt.
- Mash until smooth and well combined.
- Serve warm, garnished with a sprinkle of cinnamon.

Velvety Chocolate Avocado Mousse

Ingredients:
- 2 ripe avocados
- 1/4 cup cocoa powder
- 2-4 tablespoons honey or maple syrup (adjust to taste)

Instructions:
- Scoop the flesh of ripe avocados into a blender or food processor.
- Add cocoa powder and honey or maple syrup.
- Blend until smooth and creamy.
- Serve chilled, garnished with shaved dark chocolate or fresh berries.

Ginger-Infused Carrot Cake Puree

Ingredients:
- 2 large carrots, peeled and chopped
- 1 teaspoon freshly grated ginger
- 1 tablespoon honey or maple syrup (optional)

Instructions:
- Steam or boil the chopped carrots until soft.
- Transfer to a blender or food processor.
- Add freshly grated ginger and honey or maple syrup if desired.
- Blend until smooth and creamy.
- Serve warm or chilled, sprinkled with a pinch of ground cinnamon.

Soothing Apple Cinnamon Sauce

Ingredients:
- 2 apples, peeled, cored, and diced
- 1/2 teaspoon ground cinnamon
- 1 tablespoon lemon juice

Instructions:
- In a saucepan, combine diced apples, ground cinnamon, and lemon juice.
- Cook over medium heat, stirring occasionally, until apples are soft and tender.
- Mash the cooked apples with a fork or potato masher until desired consistency is reached.
- Serve warm as a topping for oatmeal, yogurt, or pancakes.

Minty Pea and Coconut Puree

Ingredients:
- 1 cup frozen peas, thawed
- 1/4 cup coconut milk
- 1 tablespoon fresh mint leaves, chopped

Instructions:
- In a blender or food processor, combine thawed peas, coconut milk, and chopped mint leaves.
- Blend until smooth and creamy.
- Transfer to a saucepan and warm over low heat, stirring occasionally.
- Serve warm as a side dish or chilled as a refreshing dessert.

Creamy Banana Almond Butter Puree

Ingredients:
- 2 ripe bananas
- 2 tablespoons almond butter
- 1/4 teaspoon vanilla extract

Instructions:
- Peel the ripe bananas and place them in a blender or food processor.
- Add almond butter and vanilla extract.
- Blend until smooth and creamy.
- Serve chilled as a satisfying dessert or snack.

Creamy Vanilla Bean Pear Puree

Ingredients:
- 2 ripe pears, peeled and chopped
- 1/2 teaspoon vanilla bean paste
- 1 tablespoon honey or maple syrup (optional)

Instructions:
- Steam or simmer the chopped pears until soft.
- Transfer the cooked pears to a blender or food processor.
- Add vanilla bean paste and honey or maple syrup if desired.
- Blend until smooth and creamy.
- Serve warm or chilled.

Soothing Pumpkin Spice Puree

Ingredients:
- 1 cup canned pumpkin puree
- 1/2 teaspoon pumpkin pie spice
- 2 tablespoons honey or maple syrup (optional)

Instructions:
- In a saucepan, combine canned pumpkin puree, pumpkin pie spice, and honey or maple syrup if desired.
- Cook over low heat, stirring occasionally, until heated through.
- Serve warm, sprinkled with additional pumpkin pie spice if desired.

Cozy Maple Cinnamon Butternut Squash Mash

Ingredients:
- 2 cups mashed cooked butternut squash
- 1 tablespoon maple syrup
- 1/2 teaspoon ground cinnamon

Instructions:
- In a mixing bowl, combine mashed cooked butternut squash, maple syrup, and ground cinnamon.
- Stir until well combined and smooth.
- Serve warm as a comforting side dish or dessert.

Soothing Chamomile Infused Peach Puree

Ingredients:
- 2 ripe peaches, peeled and diced
- 1/2 cup chamomile tea, brewed and cooled
- 1 tablespoon honey or maple syrup (optional)

Instructions:
- In a saucepan, combine diced peaches and brewed chamomile tea.
- Cook over medium heat until peaches are soft and tender.
- Remove from heat and let cool slightly.
- Transfer to a blender or food processor and blend until smooth.
- Add honey or maple syrup if desired, and blend again until well combined.
- Serve warm or chilled, garnished with fresh mint leaves.

HEALTHY AND TASTY SNACK RECIPES

Avocado and White Bean Dip

Ingredients:

- 1 ripe avocado
- 1 cup cooked white beans
- 1 clove garlic, minced
- 1 tablespoon lemon juice
- Salt and pepper to taste

Instructions:

- Peel and pit the avocado, then place it in a blender or food processor.
- Add the cooked white beans, minced garlic, and lemon juice to the blender.
- Blend until smooth, scraping down the sides as needed.
- Season with salt and pepper to taste.
- Transfer the dip to a serving bowl and serve with sliced vegetables or whole-grain crackers.

Sweet Potato and Carrot Hummus

Ingredients:

- 1 large sweet potato, peeled and diced
- 2 medium carrots, peeled and diced
- 1 tablespoon tahini
- 1 tablespoon olive oil
- 1 teaspoon ground cumin
- Salt and pepper to taste

Instructions:

- Steam or boil the sweet potato and carrots until tender.

- Transfer the cooked sweet potato and carrots to a blender or food processor.

- Add the tahini, olive oil, ground cumin, salt, and pepper to the blender.

- Blend until smooth, adding a splash of water if necessary to reach your desired consistency.

- Transfer the hummus to a serving bowl and sprinkle with a pinch of cumin before serving with veggie sticks or rice cakes.

Beet and Greek Yogurt Dip

Ingredients:

- 1 cup cooked beets, diced
- 1/2 cup Greek yogurt
- 1 tablespoon fresh dill, chopped
- 1 tablespoon lemon juice
- Salt and pepper to taste

Instructions:

- Place the cooked beets, Greek yogurt, fresh dill, and lemon juice in a blender or food processor.

- Blend until smooth, scraping down the sides as needed.

- Season with salt and pepper to taste.

- Transfer the dip to a serving bowl and garnish with extra dill before serving with cucumber slices or rice crackers.

Spinach and White Bean Puree

Ingredients:

- 2 cups fresh spinach leaves
- 1 cup cooked white beans
- 1 clove garlic, minced
- 2 tablespoons lemon juice
- 2 tablespoons olive oil
- Salt and pepper to taste

Instructions:

- Steam or blanch the spinach until wilted, then squeeze out any excess moisture.

- Place the cooked spinach, white beans, minced garlic, lemon juice, and olive oil in a blender or food processor.

- Blend until smooth, adding a splash of water if needed to reach your desired consistency.

- Season with salt and pepper to taste.

- Transfer the puree to a serving bowl and drizzle with a little extra olive oil before serving with rice crackers or sliced veggies.

Mango and Banana Smoothie

Ingredients:

- 1 ripe mango, peeled and diced
- 1 ripe banana
- 1/2 cup Greek yogurt
- 1/2 cup unsweetened almond milk
- 1 tablespoon honey (optional)

Instructions:

- Place the diced mango, banana, Greek yogurt, almond milk, and honey (if using) in a blender.
- Blend until smooth and creamy.
- Taste and adjust sweetness with more honey if desired.
- Pour into a glass and serve immediately.

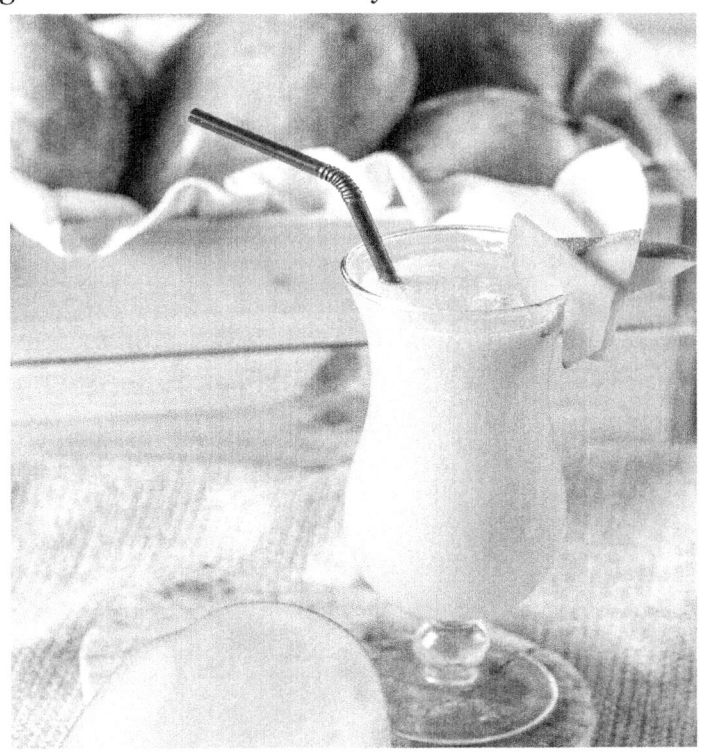

CONCLUSION

To develop a puree cookbook for adults is of great significance as far as health, well-being, and quality of life for people with varied dietary needs are concerned. Such cookbooks become indispensable to those taking care of their parents or patients who happen to be suffering from swallowing difficulties through the presentation of various ingredients that are used in coming up with new recipes and also considering nutrition.

The first advantage is that **PUREE DIET COOKBOOK FOR ADULTS** offers a range of tasty food options that are healthy which allow adults to enjoy meals regardless of strict dietary restrictions. This cookbook adds more taste to the food by using different fruits, vegetables, legumes and protein sources besides meeting the basic nutrient requirements necessary for good health.

Additionally, **PUREE DIET COOKBOOK FOR ADULTS** enhances creativity in cooking and inspires adults to try out new tastes, textures and combinations. Simple yet innovative recipes like avocado white bean dip; sweet potato carrot hummus or spinach white bean puree offer opportunities to discover the delight in preparing delicious attractive foods specific for particular diets.

Creating an inclusive puree diet recipe book is a bridge between taste and nutrition that can be used to unite the community of seniors suffering from swallowing problems among other conditions demanding modified diets. This book therefore shares recipes, advice and experiences that make adults feel part of the group in this way giving them hope that they are not alone in their path towards good health and well-being.

PUREE DIET COOKBOOK FOR ADULTS also serves as a valuable educational resource for caregivers, medical professionals or even culinary enthusiasts out there who are interested in education on matters related to pureed food. Meal planning guidance, cooking techniques and nutrition information contained in these recipes enable people to make choices based on knowledge and adapt meals for different special dietary needs.

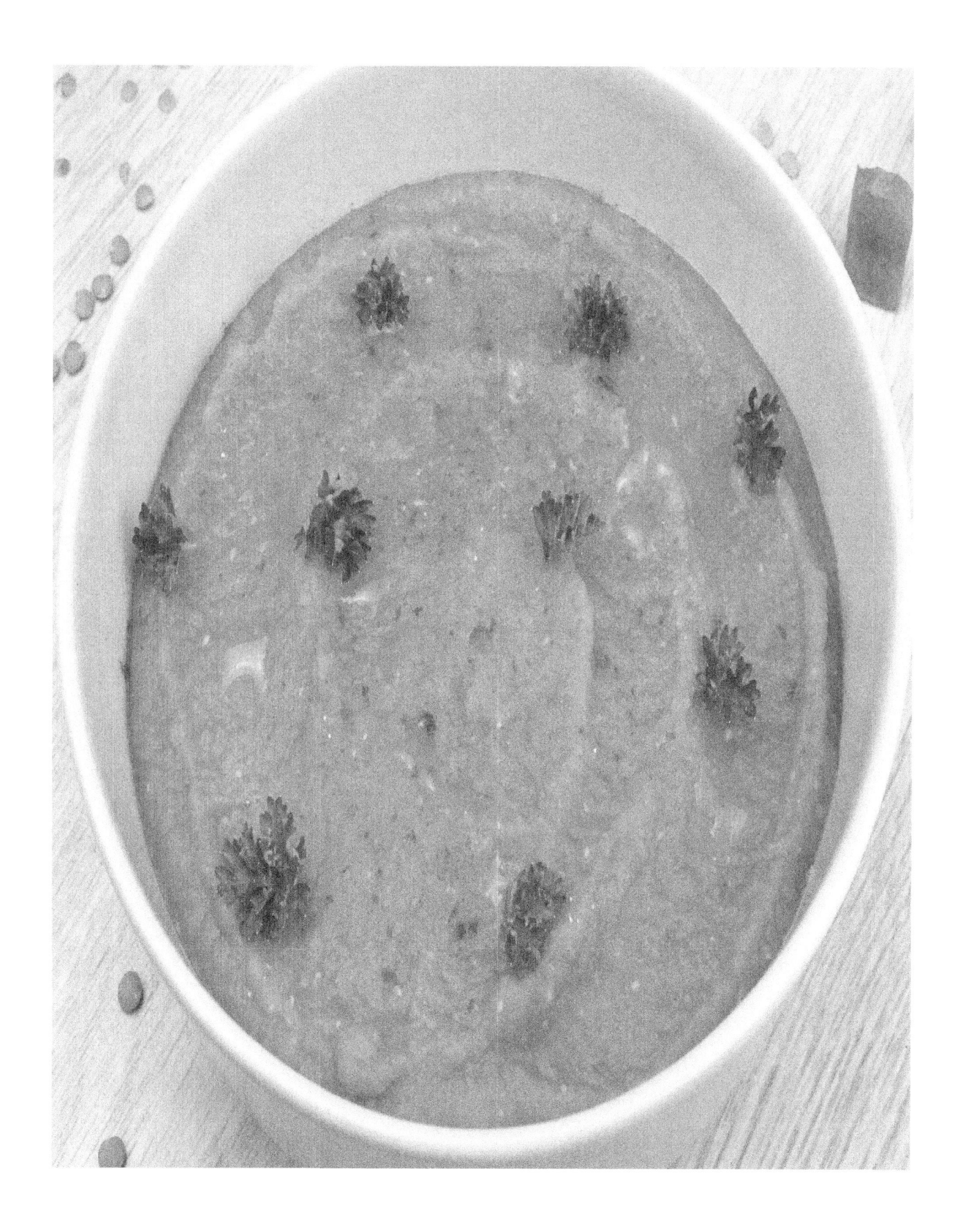

Printed in Great Britain
by Amazon